Low Carb Diet

The Fastest And Easiest Way To Rapid Fat Loss, Irrepressible Energy And Change Your Lifestyle

(Complete Guide To The Low Carb Diet Lifestyle)

Stephen Gill

TABLE OF CONTENTS

Asparagus, With Bacon And Fresh Fresh Egg 1

Bell Pepper Fresh Fresh Egg   S 3

Omelet-Stuffed Peppers 5

Broccoli And Cheese Mini Omelets.............. 7

Spiced Scrambled Fresh Fresh Egg   S 10

Sausage And Fresh Egg   Breakfast Bites.. 12

Skillet... 14

Ground Beef With Sliced Bell Peppers 16

Raspberry Shake... 18

Keto-Omelet... 19

Diet Bread 21

Fresh Egg   And Bacon................................. 23

Cajun Cauliflower Hash............................... 25

- Crunchy Cereal Mix 27
- Cream Cheese Pumpkin Pancake 29
- Skillet Baked Fresh Fresh Eggs.................. 31
- Breakfast Sausages 35
- Celery Root Hash Browns 37
- Scrambled Tofu... 39
- Spaghetti Squash 41
- Chicken Curry Salad 43
- Fresh Egg Salad... 45
- Tofu Salad 47
- Sirloin Steak Salad With Gorgonzola And Pine Nuts.. 49
- Caper And Lemon Salad 52
- Caesar Salad.. 54
- Keto Cobb Salad.. 56
- Fresh Egg Salad... 58
- Spinach And Apple Salad 60
- Mushrooms & Salad With Goat Cheese 62

Keto Warm Salad For Kale 64

Cranberry Snack Bars Sweet Potato 66

Ingredients 66

Blueberry Muffins Chocolate Muffins 68

Shroom Iced Mocha No Tension 71

Savoury Indian Pancake 72

Scrambled Fresh Fresh Egg S With Salmon 74

Tropical Smoothie Boiler 76

Smoked Salmon And Spinach Breakfast ... 77

Prosciutto-Wrapped Avocado Fresh Fresh Egg 80

Smoked Salmon Fresh Fresh Egg S Benedict 83

Chocolate Breakfast Milkshake 86

Cherry Muffins 88

Shakshuka 90

Nourishing Turmeric Scramble 93

Artichoke Ricotta Flatbread 95

Grilled Sauerkraut, Hummus, And Avocado Sandwich 98

Spinach And Feta Frittata 100

Quinoa And Citrus Salad 102

Lentil, Beetroot, And Hazelnut Salad 104

Cauliflower Steak With Beans And Tomatoes 106

Lettuce Wraps With Smoked Trout 110

Baked Sweet Potatoes With Tahini Sauce 113

Roasted Salmon With Smoky Chickpeas & Greens 116

Mediterranean Chicken Quinoa Bowl 119

Tomato, Cucumber & White-Bean Salad With Basil Vinaigrette 121

Pesto Pasta Salad 123

Slow-Cooker Mediterranean Stew 125

Salmon Potatoes 128

Mediterranean Ravioli With Artichokes & Olives.. 131

Mushrooms Of Greek Stuffed Portobello 133

Asparagus, With Bacon And Fresh Fresh Egg

Ingredients:

- slices of bacon, diced
- 2 fresh egg
- 2 oz asparagus

Seasoning:

- 2 tsp ground black pepper
- 2 tsp salt

Directions:

1 Take a skillet pan, place it over medium heat, add bacon, and cook for 10 minutes until crispy.
2 Transfer cooked bacon to a plate, then add asparagus into the pan and cook for 6 minutes until tender-crisp.

3   Crack the fresh egg over the cooked asparagus, season with salt and black pepper, then switch heat to medium-low level and cook for 2 minutes until the fresh egg white has set.
4   Chop the cooked bacon slices, sprinkle over fresh egg and asparagus and serve.

Bell Pepper Fresh Fresh Egg   s

Ingredients:

- 2 fresh fresh egg   s
- 2 green bell pepper

Seasoning:

- 2 tsp coconut oil
- 2 tsp salt
- 2 tsp ground black pepper

Directions:

1 Prepare pepper rings, and for this, cut out two slices from the pepper, about ¼-inch, and reserve remaining bell pepper for later use.
2 Take a skillet pan, place it over medium heat, grease it with oil, place pepper

rings in it, and then crack an fresh egg into each ring.

3. Season fresh fresh eggs with salt and black pepper, cook for 10 minutes, or until fresh fresh eggs have cooked to the desired level.

4. Transfer fresh fresh eggs to a plate and serve.

Omelet-Stuffed Peppers

Ingredients:

- 2slices of bacon, chopped, cooked
- 2 tbsp grated parmesan cheese
- 2 fresh green bell pepper, halved, cored
- 2 fresh fresh egg s

Seasoning:

- 2 tsp ground black pepper
- 2 tsp salt

Directions:

1 Turn on the oven, then set it to 820 degrees F, and let preheat.
2 Then take a baking dish, pour in 2 tbsp water, place bell pepper halved in it, cut-side up, and bake for 2 0 minutes.

3 Meanwhile, crack fresh fresh eggs in a bowl, add chopped bacon and cheese, season with salt and black pepper, and whisk until combined.
4 After 6 minutes of baking time, remove baking dish from the oven, evenly fill the peppers with fresh egg mixture and continue baking for 2 6 to 20 minutes until fresh fresh eggs have set.
5 Serve.

Broccoli And Cheese Mini Omelets

Ingredients

- 2 cup grated cheese of your choice
- 2 teaspoon of olive oil
- A dash of salt and pepper
- Cooking spray or a small amount of butter
- 6 fresh fresh fresh egg s
- cup fresh egg whites
- cups of broccoli florets
- cup shredded cheddar cheese

Directions

1 Start by preheating your oven to 680 degrees Fahrenheit. While the oven is preheating, steam the broccoli florets in a small amount of water for about 6 to 8 minutes. Once removed and strained,

they should crumble into smaller pieces. Add them along with the olive oil, salt, and pepper into a mixing bowl. Mix thoroughly.

2 Spray a cupcake or muffin tin with cooking spray or line with butter.

3 Spread the broccoli mixture along the bottoms of the muffin cups.

4 In a medium bowl, beat the fresh egg whites and fresh fresh egg s together. Add the grated cheese of your choice. Pour this over the broccoli mixture, until the cup is about 1/2 full. Top the mini omelets with cheddar cheese and bake for about 20 minutes. The edges should be brown and the tops fluffy. You can serve immediately or store them for future meals.

Spiced Scrambled Fresh Fresh Egg   S

Ingredients

- 2 tablespoon of milk
- 2 handful of diced fresh tomato   es
- Coriander leaves
- 2 tablespoon of butter
- 2 small fresh onion   (chopped)
- red chili pepper (chopped)
- fresh fresh egg   s (beaten)

Directions

1. Start by softening the chopped fresh onion   and chili in a frying pan with the tablespoon of butter.
2. Once the vegetables have softened, add the fresh fresh egg   s and a tablespoon or splash of milk.

3 Gently scramble the fresh fresh eggs as they cook. When the fresh fresh eggs are almost scrambled, add the diced fresh tomatoes and a few coriander leaves. Serve while still hot.

Sausage And Fresh Egg Breakfast Bites

Ingredients

- 2 fresh fresh egg   s
- A small handful of parsley
- handful of dark greens (spinach, kale, beet greens, or Swiss chard)
- 2 cups of crumbled sausage (uncooked)

Directions

1 Preheat your oven to 620 degrees Fahrenheit. Slice the greens into thin strips. If you are using kale, you will need to remove the stems. Sauté a small amount of olive oil or butter over medium heat in a fresh skillet. Add the

crumbled sausage. Once the sausage is mostly cooked, turn off the heat.

2   In a fresh mixing bowl, whisk the fresh fresh fresh egg   s parsley, dark greens, and sausage together. Pour this mixture into a greased 8x8 pan. Bake for 20 to 4 0 minutes, or until the tops are crispy. Allow to cool for several minutes before cutting into squares.

Skillet

Ingredients

- 2 cups cauliflower (grated)
- 2 tablespoon butter
- 6 tablespoon extra-virgin olive oil
- 2 whole fresh fresh eggs
- 6 fresh egg whites
- 2 cup shredded sharp cheddar cheese
- green onions (chopped)
- strips of bacon (cooked and crumbled)

Directions

1. Preheat your broiler with your oven rack positioned in the center slot. Heat the oil and butter in an oven-proof skillet over medium heat. Add the cauliflower and season with a dash of salt and pepper. Sauté until golden brown. This should take about 6 to 8 minutes.

2 In a fresh mixing bowl, add the fresh fresh fresh egg s fresh egg whites, 2 cup of cheese, fresh onions, and bacon. Mix thoroughly with a fork.

3 Once the cauliflower is cooked, spread the cauliflower to form an even layer along the bottom of the skillet.

4 Pour the fresh egg mixture over the cauliflower. Use a spatula to smooth the mixture. Cook until the sides are set. This should take about 10 minutes . Add the remaining 2 cup of cheddar cheese. Place the skillet in your oven and broil until the cheese is bubbly – about 6 to 10 minutes . Allow to cool for 35minutes before cutting and serving.

Ground Beef With Sliced Bell Peppers

Ingredients

- 2 tablespoon coconut oil (or olive oil)
- 2 handful of spinach
- 2 pound of ground beef
- Salt and pepper (to taste)
- 2 red bell pepper (sliced)
- 2 small fresh onion

Directions

1. First, cut the fresh onion into small pieces.
2. Place some coconut oil or olive oil in a frying pan.
3. Fry the chopped fresh onion for about two minutes.
4. Add the ground beef and season with some salt and pepper.

5 After cooking the meat for several minutes, add the spinach. Continue stirring until the meat is fully cooked. Serve with a sliced bell pepper. This serves one person, but you could easily double the recipe to make two servings.

Raspberry Shake

Ingredients:

- 6   tbsp of cream
- 2 tbsp of vanilla whey protein powder
- 2 cup of fresh raspberries
- 2 cup of unsweetened almond milk

Directions:

1. Pour the almond milk into the blender along with the cream.
2. Add the protein powder and raspberries.
3. Blend all the ingredients into a nutritious smoothie.

Keto-Omelet

Ingredients:

- 2 cup of spinach
- 2 small onion
- 2 small fresh tomato
- 2 tsp of basil
- Olive oil
- 2 tbsp of unsweetened almond milk
- 2 fresh egg whites
- 2 fresh egg yolk

Directions:

1. First, finely chop the onion, fresh tomato and spinach.
2. In another bowl, whisk the fresh egg whites and single yolk with the almond milk. It should become smooth and frothy.

3 Mix the vegetables and fresh egg mixture with some basil.
4 Pour some olive oil into a skillet and let it heat.
5 Then cook your healthy omelet!

Diet Bread

Ingredients:

- 2 tsp of Celtic sea salt
- 6 tbsp of oat fiber
- 6 tbsp of psyllium husk powder

- 2 fresh egg
- 2 cup of hot water
- 280 ml of unsweetened coconut milk
- 6 tbsp of butter
- 2 cup of almond flour
- 2 tsp of baking powder

Directions:

1. In a bowl, mix the almond flour with the husk powder, salt and baking powder into an even mixture.
2. Over low heat, place the solids of the chilled coconut milk and butter. Then

remove from heat and whisk well. Whisk the fresh egg into this.

3 Mix the dry mixture with the wet mixture. Beat it into a firm dough. Break this into small parts.

4 Boil the water and pour it into the bowl of dough. Stir it well.

5 Now scoop out your dough and place on the baking sheets. Keep each ball a little apart.

6 Let the bread bake in the oven for about 8 0 minutes and then let it cool before serving.

Fresh Egg And Bacon

Ingredients

- 6 slices bacon
- Salt to taste
- Pepper to taste
- Fresh tomato circles to serve
- 6 fresh fresh fresh fresh egg s beaten
- 2 cup full fat cream
- 2 tablespoon butter

Directions:

1. Preheat the oven to 680 Fahrenheit
2. Place the bacon on the baking tray such that they are not overlapping and have enough space.
3. Place them in the oven for 20 to 30 minutes or until completely crispy.

4 Meanwhile, place the fresh fresh eggs in a bowl and beat it.
5 Add in the cream, salt and pepper and beat until well combined.
6 Add the butter to a pan and once it heats, add in the fresh fresh eggs and allow it to scramble.
7 Place the bacon strips on the side of the plate and place the fresh fresh eggs on another corner.
8 Add in the fresh tomato slices and serve hot!

Cajun Cauliflower Hash

Ingredients:

- 2 teaspoons Cajun seasoning
- ounce shaved red pastrami, chopped into 2 -inch slices
- 2 green pepper, chopped into 2 inch pieces
- A few fresh fresh fresh egg s fried sunny side up
- 6 tablespoons olive oil or ghee
- 2 onion, chopped into 2 inch pieces
- 6 tablespoons garlic, minced
- 2 pounds frozen cauliflower, steamed, chopped into small, squeezed of all moisture

Directions:

1. Place a skillet over medium heat. Add oil. When the oil is heated, add onions. Sauté until the onions are translucent.
2. Add garlic and sauté for a couple of minutes until the garlic is fragrant.
3. Add cauliflower and sauté until it starts getting brown.
4. Add Cajun seasoning. Stir well.
5. Add pastrami and green pepper. Cook until thoroughly heated.
6. Transfer into individual serving bowls.
7. Top with fresh fresh egg   s . Sprinkle some more Cajun seasoning over it.

Crunchy Cereal Mix

Ingredients:

- Unsweetened milk of your choice
- Low carb fruits of your choice, chopped
- Nuts of your choice
- 6 cups flaked coconut
- 2 teaspoons ground cinnamon
- Stevia to taste (optional)

Directions:

1. Line a cookie sheet with parchment paper. Spread the coconut flakes over the cookie sheet.
2. Roast in the oven for about 6 minutes. Keep a watch over the oven. Mix the flakes in between a couple of times and roast until light brown.

3. Remove from the oven. Leave it aside to cool. Sprinkle cinnamon powder. It will turn out crunchy in a while.
4. Serve with milk, stevia and fruits and nuts.
5. In case you want to store it, transfer the cooled coconut flakes into an airtight container. Add nuts. Mix well and store it in a cool dry place.

Cream Cheese Pumpkin Pancake

Ingredients:

For the pumpkin butter:

- 6 tablespoons butter, unsalted
- 2 teaspoon stevia
- 2 tablespoon 2 00% pumpkin

For the pancakes:

- 6 ounces cream cheese
- 6 fresh egg
- 6 tablespoons coconut flour
- 2 tablespoon pumpkin pie spice blend
- 6 tablespoons butter

Directions:

1. To make the pumpkin butter: Place butter and pumpkin in a microwavable dish. Mix well. Microwave for 35seconds on high. Mix well. If not smooth, microwave again for 35seconds.
2. When the pumpkin butter is smooth, add stevia.
3. To make the pancakes: Add cream cheese, fresh fresh fresh egg s coconut flour and pumpkin pie spice to the blender. Blend until smooth. Transfer into a bowl.
4. Place a nonstick pan over medium heat. Add 2 -tablespoon butter.
5. When the butter melts and begins to brown, pour about 2 of the batter. Swirl the pan a bit so that the pancake spreads.
6. Cook until the bottom side is golden brown. Flip sides and cook the other side too.
7. Repeat steps 6 and 6 with the remaining batter.

8. Place a little of the pumpkin butter on the pancake and serve.

Skillet Baked Fresh Fresh Eggs

Ingredients:

- 6 tablespoons leek, chopped, white and pale green part only
- 6 tablespoons scallions, chopped, white and pale green parts only
- 6 ounces fresh spinach, rinsed
- 6 teaspoons fresh lemon juice
- 2 fresh fresh fresh egg s
- 6 teaspoon crushed red pepper flakes
- 2 teaspoon paprika
- 2 teaspoons fresh oregano, chopped
- 2 cup plain Greek yogurt
- 6 cloves garlic, halved

- 6 Kosher salt to taste
- 6 tablespoons unsalted butter, divided
- 6 tablespoons olive oil

Directions:

1. To a small bowl, add yogurt, garlic and a pinch of salt. Mix well and keep aside.
2. Place a skillet over medium heat. Add butter. When the butter is heated, add leeks and scallion.
3. Lower the heat. Cook until softened.
4. Add spinach, salt and lemon juice.
5. Raise the heat to medium high. Sauté for a few minutes until the spinach is wilted.
6. Transfer the contents to a fresh ovenproof dish. Do not add the excess liquid, which is present in the spinach mixture.
7. Make 6 wells in the mixture.
8. Gently break an fresh egg into each of the wells.
9. Place the dish in a preheated oven. Bake at 6 00 degree F until the fresh fresh egg s are set.
10. Place a small saucepan over medium low heat. Add the remaining butter. When the

butter melts, add the yogurt mixture and a pinch of salt. Cook for a few seconds and add oregano. Cook for 20-50 seconds. Discard the garlic halves.

11 Pour the yogurt mixture over the fresh fresh eggs and serve.

Breakfast Sausages

Ingredients:

- 2 fresh green bell pepper, chopped into 2 inch pieces
- 2 fresh red bell pepper, chopped, chopped into 2 inch pieces
- 2 fresh yellow bell pepper, chopped, chopped into 2 inch pieces
- 2 fresh orange bell pepper, chopped, chopped into 2 inch pieces
- 6 teaspoons olive oil
- Spike seasoning to taste or any other seasoning of your choice
- Freshly ground black pepper to taste
- 2 ounces turkey breakfast sausage links
- 2 cup low fat mozzarella, grated

Directions:

1. Place the peppers in a greased baking dish. Add 2 teaspoons of oil over the peppers. Mix well.
2. Sprinkle spike seasoning and pepper powder.
3. Bake in a preheated oven at 8 0 0 degree F for about 20 minutes.
4. Meanwhile, place a nonstick pan over medium heat. Add the remaining oil. When the oil is heated, add the sausages and cook until well browned all over.
5. Remove and place on your cutting board. When cool enough to handle, chop the sausages into about 2-inch pieces.
6. Add the sausages to the baking dish and bake along with the peppers for about 6 -8 minutes.
7. Remove from the oven. Sprinkle cheese over it. Place it back in the oven.
8. Broil for a couple of minutes until the cheese is melted. Serve immediately.

Celery Root Hash Browns

Ingredients:

- 6 celery roots, peeled, grated
- 2 tablespoons coconut oil or ghee
- Salt to taste
- Pepper to taste
- Fresh tomato salsa to serve

Directions:

1. Mix salt and pepper to the celery root.
2. Place a pan over medium high heat. Add oil. When the oil is heated, add the grated celery root. Spread it all over the pan to make one fresh one or else make smaller sized ones. Smaller sized ones can be made in batches.
3. When the bottom side is cooked and golden brown, flip sides and cook the other side, too.

4 Chop into wedges.
5 Serve with fresh tomato salsa and scrambled fresh fresh eggs .

Scrambled Tofu

Ingredients:

- 2 teaspoon red chili flakes
- 2 cup cheddar cheese, shredded (optional)
- 2 tablespoons olive oil
- 2 bunches green fresh onions, chopped
- cans peeled, diced fresh tomatoes along with the juice
- 2 packages (35ounce each) firm silken tofu, drained, mashed
- 2 teaspoon ground turmeric
- Salt to taste
- Pepper powder to taste

Directions:

1 Place a skillet over medium heat. Add oil. When the oil is heated, add green

onions. Sauté until the green onions are tender.
2. Add turmeric, salt and pepper. Sauté for a couple of minutes.
3. Add tofu and fresh tomatoes along with the juice. Mix well.
4. Lower heat and let it heat thoroughly. Sprinkle cheddar cheese if desired, and serve.

Spaghetti Squash

Ingredients:

- 2 cup of cream
- 2 fresh egg yolks
- 2 cup of grated cheese
- 2 tsp of garlic paste
- Salt
- 2 fresh spaghetti squash
- 6 tbsp of butter
- 2 cup of baked ham

Directions:

1. Cut the squash up and remove the pulp as well as the seeds from the inside.
2. Bake the squash at about 6 20 degrees and then let it cool.
3. Cut out the strands using a fork.
4. Place a saucepan over medium heat. Melt the butter on this.

5. Sauté the chopped ham on the butter for a couple of minutes.
6. Whisk the fresh egg yolk with the cream and add to the pan.
7. Stir in the garlic and cheese. Let this all cook for a few minutes.
8. Then add the squash and mix well till you get a creamy consistency.
9. Serve hot.

Chicken Curry Salad

Ingredients:

- 2 tbsp of butter
- 2 fresh egg yolk
- 2 tbsp of mayonnaise
- 2 tsp of lemon juice
- A sprinkle of salt
- 2 tsp of curry powder
- 2 cup of cooked chicken
- 2 cup of celery
- A handful of almonds

Directions:

1. Place a skillet over low heat and melt the butter. Then remove it from heat.
2. Whisk the butter with the fresh egg yolk and then add the mayonnaise. Whisk well.

3. Add the lemon juice, curry powder and salt and whisk it all together. Keep this as your salad dressing.
4. Mix the dressing with the diced chicken. Add some celery and sliced almonds. Your salad is ready!

Fresh Egg Salad

Ingredients:

- Pinch of ground mustard
- 2 tbsp of minced onion
- Sprinkle of black pepper
- Pinch of salt
- 6 fresh eggs
- 2 cup of mayonnaise
- 2 tbsp of butter

Directions:

1. First cook the fresh fresh eggs in a pot of boiling water for about 35minutes.
2. Put the fresh fresh eggs into cold water and let it cool.
3. Then peel and chop the cooked fresh fresh egg s .
4. Mix the fresh fresh egg s with the mayonnaise, butter, mustard, and onion.

5   Add the salt and pepper to taste.
6   It can be kept in the fridge till you want to serve!

Tofu Salad

Ingredients:

- 2 tsp of minced garlic
- 2 tsp of rice vinegar
- 2 tbsp of lemon juice
- 250 gms of Chinese cabbage
- 2 tbsp of cilantro
- 2 tbsp of virgin coconut oil
- 2 tbsp of peanut butter
- 6 drops of liquid stevia
- 250 gms firm tofu
- 2 tbsp of soy sauce
- 2 tsp of sesame oil
- 2 tbsp of water

Directions:

1 First, press and dry out your tofu.

2. In a bowl, mix 2 tsp sesame oil and soy sauce with the vinegar and garlic. Add 2 tsp of lemon juice. This is your marinade.
3. Pour the marinade along with the tofu into a Ziploc bag and leave it for an hour.
4. Then bake the chopped tofu for about 80 minutes at 640 degrees or so.
5. While the tofu is baking, make the rest of your salad.
6. Chop up the cilantro and mix with the remaining ingredients except the Chinese cabbage and lime juice.
7. Slice up the Chinese cabbage.
8. Just before adding the tofu, mix the sliced cabbage and lemon juice into the dressing.
9. Then add the tofu and mix.

Sirloin Steak Salad With Gorgonzola And Pine Nuts

Ingredients:

- 6 teaspoon fresh rosemary
- 2 tablespoon red wine vinegar
- 2 teaspoon Dijon mustard or to taste
- 2 clove garlic, minced
- cups mixed baby greens
- 2 tablespoons pine nuts, toasted
- ounce Gorgonzola cheese, crumbled
- 2 sirloin steak of about a pound and an inch thick
- 2 tablespoons olive oil
- Kosher salt to taste
- Freshly ground black pepper to taste

Directions:

1. Apply the steak with 2 /2-tablespoon olive oil. Rub well. Season with salt and pepper.
2. Take a little of the rosemary and rub it over the steak. Leave aside for an hour at room temperature or refrigerate for at least 6 hours, uncovered.
3. If you refrigerate it, then remove from the oven about 8 0 minutes before you grill it.
4. Prepare a grill, either a charcoal grill or gas grill or a grill pan placed over high heat.
5. Place the steak on the grill rack of whatever Directions: you are using to grill. Grill for a couple of minutes. Flip sides and grill the other side for a couple of minutes or until done.

6 Transfer onto a plate. Cover it loosely for a few minutes. When cool enough to handle, cut the steak across the grains.
7 Meanwhile, add vinegar, mustard, garlic, salt and pepper to a bowl. Whisk constantly. Whisking constantly, pour the remaining oil in a thin stream. Continue whisking until the mixture is emulsified.
8 To serve: Place the greens in a serving bowl. Place the steak slices over it. Sprinkle pine nuts and Gorgonzola cheese. Sprinkle the dressing and serve immediately.

Caper And Lemon Salad

Ingredients:

- 2 Juice of a lemon or to taste
- 2 teaspoon lemon zest, grated
- 2 cup canned capers, drained, rinsed
- stalks celery, chopped
- 2 teaspoon fresh dill, chopped
- 2tablespoons extra virgin olive oil
- 6 pounds salmon fillet
- Salt to taste
- 2 Pepper to taste

Directions:

1. Season the salmon with salt and pepper and bake in a preheated oven at 680 degree F for 35minutes or until the salmon is flaky.

2. Transfer the salmon to a serving bowl. Add lemon juice, lemon zest, capers, celery, dill and olive oil and toss.
3. Place in the refrigerator until use.

Caesar Salad

Ingredients:

- 2 ounces pork rinds, chopped in small pieces
- 2 cup parmesan cheese, shaved for garnish
- 2 cup homemade mayonnaise - refer to Chapter 6
- 8 anchovy filets
- 6 garlic cloves
- 2 cup parmesan, grated
- 35 whole leaves of romaine hearts, rinsed, pat dried

Directions:

1. Add anchovies, garlic and parmesan.
2. Blend again on low until the mixture is well combined and of smooth texture.

3. Lay the lettuce leaves on individual plates. Spread a little of the mayonnaise over the leaves.
4. Divide the pork pieces amongst the plates.
5. Serve garnished with parmesan.

Keto Cobb Salad

Ingredients:

For the dressing:

- 2 teaspoons lemon juice
- 2 teaspoons Dijon mustard
- 2 clove garlic, minced
- Salt to taste
- 2 Pepper powder to taste
- 2 tablespoons olive oil
- 2 tablespoons apple cider vinegar

For the salad:
- Cooking spray
- 2 cup ham, chopped into cubes
- 8 cherry fresh tomato es
- 2 cup blue cheese, shredded
- hard-boiled fresh fresh fresh egg s sliced

- 6   cups romaine lettuce chopped
- 2 avocado, peeled, pitted, diced
- 3 slices turkey bacon

Directions:

1 Mix together all the ingredients of the dressing. Whisk well and keep aside.
2 Place a pan over medium heat. Spray with cooking spray. Add the ham and cook for about 6 minutes. Remove from heat and keep aside.
3 Place the lettuce at the bottom of a fresh salad bowl.
4 Lay the fresh tomato   es, avocado, blue cheese, ham, fresh fresh egg   s and ban in rows.
5 Sprinkle the dressing and serve.

Fresh Egg Salad

Ingredients:

- 2 teaspoon Dijon mustard
- 2 teaspoon lemon juice
- Salt to taste
- Pepper to taste
- Lettuce leaves to serve
- 2 fresh fresh fresh egg s hard-boiled, chopped into small pieces
- 2

Directions:

1. Mix together the fresh fresh fresh eggs mayonnaise, mustard, lemon juice, salt and pepper in a bowl.
2. Adjust the seasonings if necessary.
3. Serve over lettuce leaves.

Spinach And Apple Salad

Ingredients:

For the salad:
- 8 cups baby spinach leaves, rinsed
- 2 cup red onion, thinly sliced
- 2 cup blue cheese, crumbled
- 2 apple, cored, cut into small cubes

For the dressing:

- 2 cup cold-pressed olive oil
- 2 cup red wine vinegar
- 2 cloves garlic, minced
- 2 cup feta cheese, crumbled
- 8 slices thin bacon, cooked, crumbled to serve

Directions:

1. To make the dressing: Blend together all the ingredients of the dressing until smooth. Transfer into a glass bowl. Add bacon and mix well.
2. Place the spinach leaves over a fresh serving platter. Lay the apple pieces over the spinach.
3. Drizzle the dressing all over the salad. Toss and serve.

Mushrooms & Salad With Goat Cheese

Ingredients:

- ounces of sliced cremini mushrooms.
- ounces of spring mix
- Pepper and salt
- ounceof cooked, crumbled bacon.
- tablespoon of balsamic vinegar
- 2   ounce of crumbled goat cheese.
- 2   tablespoon of butter
- 2   tablespoon of olive oil

Direction:

1 . Heat the butter in a medium saucepan.

2. Sautee the spores before the mushrooms are tender and brown. To try, season with salt and pepper.
3. . Meanwhile, put the salad greens in a bowl. Complete with bacon and goat's crumbled cheese.
4. Mix them into the salad until the mushrooms are finished.
5. . In a small cup, mix together the olive oil and the balsamic vinegar. Place your salad on top and eat.

Keto Warm Salad For Kale

Ingredients:

For Warm Salad

- 3 ounces of feta cheese
- 1 ounces of kale
- Pepper and salt
- 2 tablespoons of butter

For Dressing

- 2 teaspoon ofdijon mustard
- 1 teaspoon of garlic
- 5 tablespoons of whipping cream
- 2 mteaspoon of mayonnaise

Direction:

1. . Mix together the heavy cream, mayonnaise, mustard from Dijon, and the garlic until smooth. And put aside.

2. Rinse and cut the kale into bits that are bite-sized. Dispose of the stem.
3. . Apply the butter over medium heat to a plate. When the kale is heavy, add it to the pan and cook quickly until it turns dark brown. 2 -2 minutes usually.
4. Set the cooked kale in a tub. Cover it with dressing and feta cheese. To try, season with salt and pepper.

Cranberry Snack Bars Sweet Potato

Ingredients

- 2 cup of almond meal
- 3 -third cup of coconut flour
- 2 and 1 t baking soda
- 2 cup of fresh cranberries
- 2 and 1 cups of purée sweet potato
- 2 -quarter cup of water
- tin of melted coconut oil.
- tin of maple syrup
- 3 fresh fresh eggs

Directions:

1 Heat the oven to a temperature of 480 ° F.

2. Mix the coconut flour, crushed potatoes, water, coconut oil mixed with maple syrup and fresh fresh egg s into a fresh mixing pot. Turn the mixture until combined.
3. Sift the almond meal, coconut flour and baked soda together in another bowl and blend them well.
4. In the sweet potato mixture add the dry ingredients and combine properly.
5. Grease a 15 -inch baker pot and cocoon oil and parchment paper underneath the jar.
6. Move the batter to the prepared mixer, use a wet spatula to lighten the surface and fill the corners. Place the pulp on the end.
7. Bake for 4 0-45 minutes just until the center toothpick is clean. Cool before slicing into squares and being removed from the oven.

Blueberry Muffins
Chocolate Muffins

Ingredients:

- 2 teaspoon of baking powder
- 2 tablespoon of coconut flour
- 1 cup of almond flour
- 1 cup of unsweetened almond milk
- 2 -quarter cup of fresh blueberries
- tablespoon of dark chocolate chips
- 3 fresh fresh fresh egg s
- 2 small ripped avocado pear
- 2 -third cup of coconut sugar
- 2 -quarter teaspoon of salt
- 2 -quarter cup of raw cacao powder plus 2 tablespoon

Directions:

1 Heat the oven to 500 degrees F. Prepare a muffin pan or cocoon oil grate with muffin liners.
2 In a blender, put the fresh egg s, avocado, sugar and salt with 2 tablespoon of cacao powder. Combine strongly before avocado is completely disintegrated, so that the mixture is smooth.
3 Sift 2 /4 cup of chocolate, baking powder, chocolate flour and almond meal together in a small dish.
4 Fill in the liquid combination with almond milk and gently insert into dry ingredients. Mixing-do n't mix together! Blend before mixing!
5 Fold in chops and blueberries.
6 Shift the flour to the prepared muffin tin and uniformly split the flour into 15 cavities.

7 Bake for 30 minutes or till when it comes out clear with a toothpick inserted into the muffin core.
8 Take out the muffins from the jar and refrigerate into a wire baking rack.
9 Store for 2 week in the refrigerator, or for up to 2 month in the fridge.

Shroom Iced Mocha No Tension

Ingredients:

- 2 teaspoon of coconut oil
- 1 tablespoon of raw cacao powder
- 1 cup of unsweetened almond milk
- Handful of ice cubes
- packet of Mushroom Coffee with Lion's Mane and 5 Sigmatic (chaga)
- 9 oz of hot water

Direction:

1. Add hot water to 5 Sigmatic package. Remove powder to dissolve and allow to cool for 2 minutes.
2. Replace the coconut oil and cacao powder until it has dissolved.
3. Pour the almond milk over the chocolate, add ice and drink!

Savoury Indian Pancake

INGREDIENTS

- teaspoon of salt, regulate to taste
- 1 teaspoon of Kashmiri Chili Powder
- -quarter teaspoon of Turmeric Powder
- 2 -quarter teaspoon of freshly ground black pepper
- 1 chopped of red onion
- 2 handful of chopped cilantro leaves
- 2 Serrano minced pepper
- 1 inch of grated ginger.
- Oil or fat of choice, use much to shallow fry
- 1 cup of Almond Flour
- 1 cup of Tapioca Flour
- 2 cup of Coconut Milk, canned and full fat

Directions:

1. . Put in a cup almond flour, tapioca flour, coconut milk and spices-blend together.
2. Stir in the cabbage, coriander, serrano pepper and ginger.
3. Pancakes cook!
4. . Heat a sauté pan on low-medium heat, add sufficient oil / fat to cover the pan, then spill 2 /4 cup of batter over the pan. Spread the mixture over the saucepan.
5. Fry this for about 4 -4 minutes per side – drizzle a little more oil over the pancake before flipping it. (Stoves differ, which cook until golden brown on both sides).
6. . Repeat until the batter is finished- keep adding oil if appropriate.
7. Feed with vegetable chutney or paleo ketchup.

Scrambled Fresh Fresh Egg S With Salmon

Ingredients:

- 2 tbsp. coconut milk;
- Fresh chives, finely chopped;
- fresh egg s;
- slices smoked salmon, chopped;

Directions:

1 Whisk up the fresh egg s, coconut milk, and fresh chives in a cup. Tasteful season.
2 Melt some fat in a pan and then add the fresh egg s.
3 Scramble about the fresh fresh egg s as you prepare.
4 Add the smoked salmon and cook for 2 to 2 minutes until the fresh fresh egg s begin to settle.

5 Serve over sprayed with far more chives.

Tropical Smoothie Boiler

INGREDIENTS

- 1 of banana
- spoonful of chia
- 2 quarter tablespoon of turmeric
- 2   cup of orange juice
- 2   cup of frozen pineapple
- 2   cup of frozen mango

Direction:

1. In the order specified, apply all the ingredients to a blender.
2. Blend until soft and shiny.
3. If the mixture is too thick you may need to add a splash of orange juice.
4. Cover with cut mango, coconut flakes and almonds.

Smoked Salmon And Spinach Breakfast

Ingredients:

- 2 minced of garlic clove
- 1 teaspoon of onion powder
- 1 teaspoon of garlic powder
- 2 -quarter teaspoon of paprika
- 2 tablespoon of ghee
- 4 tablespoon of olive oil
- Freshly ground black pepper and Sea salt
- fresh fresh egg s
- 1 oz. of smoked salmon, sliced
- russet or sweet potatoes, peeled and diced
- 1 of sliced onion
- 1 cup of sliced mushrooms
- 3   cups of fresh baby spinach

Directions:

1. Oven preheat to 426 F.
2. Dice the potatoes, drizzle with olive oil, onions , garlic, peppers and season to taste. Dice the potatoes.
3. Place the potatoes on the bakery platter and roast in the oven for 30-50 minutes.
4. Place a pot of water on high heat and carry to boil.
5. Connect the fresh fresh egg s to the boiling water and switching off the flame, cooking for 8 to 10 minutes.
6. Drain the water over the fresh fresh egg s and run cold water; remove the fresh egg s, and put aside.
7. Dissolve the ghee with medium to high heat, and add garlic and onion.
8. Cook for 5 to 10 minutes, then add the chopped mushrooms.

9. Season all to taste, and simmer for 10 to 15 minutes, until everything is smooth.
10. Attach the spinach, and simmer for 5 to 5 minutes until wilted.

Prosciutto-Wrapped Avocado Fresh Fresh Egg

Ingredients:

- 2 tablespoon of olive oil
- Salt and pepper
- Sliced tomato, for garnish
- Chopped parsley, for garnish
- 2 ripe avocados
- 2 fresh fresh egg s
- slices of prosciutto

Directions:

1. Boil a small pot of water using low heat until a gentle simmer is achieved.
2. Line an undersized mixing bowl with a plastic wrap that is food safe and massage a modest olive oil on it.

3 Break inside the lined bowl an fresh egg , then tie a knot by pulling the both sides of the wrap as 2 . Put the already wrapped fresh fresh egg inside the boiling water for up to 4 mins. Do the same to the other fresh egg .

4 Take out the fresh fresh egg s from inside the water and put it on a plate. Then gently part the fresh fresh egg s by cutting the wraps open. Set the fresh fresh egg s apart from each other

5 Set up the prosciutto slices by levelling them. This can be achieved by using a knife back.

6 Divide the avocado into 3 and take out the outermost skin. hollow out the centre of the avocado making it to be the equal size as with the already poached fresh egg . Cautiously place the fresh fresh egg inside the avocado and enclose it from both sides.

7 Enfold the conserved avocado firmly in prosciutto slices, setting 2

8. strips horizontally and 2 vertically. Replicate these steps to the remaining fresh egg .
9. Fry the in olive oil Using a medium heat, the prosciutto-wrapped avocado should be fried in olive oil for up to 30 minutes, commencing with the end of the bacon that is loose. Flip over frequently till all the bacon becomes crispy all over.

Smoked Salmon Fresh Fresh Egg S Benedict

INGREDIENTS

- 2 teaspoons of capers
- 2 Thinly sliced red onion
- 2 A pinch of black pepper
- 2 fresh fresh fresh egg yolks
- 2 tablespoons of water
- 3 tablespoons of butter (use ghee for Whole55 plus paleo)
- 2 teaspoons of fresh lemon juice
- A pinch of salt
- fresh fresh fresh egg s
- 3 English muffins cut into 1 (Gluten-free, if needed. See notes for Whole55 plus paleo)
- 5 tablespoons of cream cheese (neglect for Whole55 plus paleo) 4 ounces of smoked salmon (lox)

Directions:

1. .First mix the Hollandaise sauce. Attach a medium frying pan with the fresh fresh egg yolks and the water. Place the frying pan 2 inches over a medium-high portion and stir the fresh fresh egg s till they are soft and frothy. Apply the butter to the saucepan (do not put the pan on the element!) and stir till thick is the hollandaise. Mix the lemon juice as well as a sprinkle of salt and set it aside the saucepan.
2. Put a medium-sized pot of boiling water over high temperature on the burner.
3. . Toast the English muffins gently, in either a toaster or by frying them on their sliced sides in a little butter.
4. Position each mostly on serving plates, then add the cream cheese on top.
5. Split the smoked salmon among them .

6. 6 . Reduce heat as the water starts to boil, so that it simmers softly. Put the fresh fresh egg s 2 by 2 , and simmer for 5 minutes. Use a rubber spatula to take them away from the pot, and place 2 fresh fresh egg over each English muffin.
7. Pour over the fresh fresh egg s and finish the hollandaise sauce with some pieces of red onion, some capers and just a little black pepper.
8. Toss several of baby arugula with such a splash of olive oil and put the salad next to the fresh fresh egg s Benedict.

Chocolate Breakfast Milkshake

Ingredients:

- 2   tablespoon of raw cacao powder
- 1 teaspoon of vanilla extract
- 5 ice cubes
- 3 fresh of frozen organic bananas
- 2 cup of coconut milk
- 3 tablespoon of cashew butter

Directions

1. Begin by adding to your blender, the bananas and coconut milk, and pulse a few times.
2. Attach the cashew butter, cacao powder and mint, then pulse a few more times.
3. Put ice, then mix until smooth. Add additional ice cubes or more coconut

milk if required to ensure consistency for a milkshake.

Cherry Muffins

Ingredients:

- 2 quarter cup of maple syrup or 1 teaspoon of stevia liquid 3 teaspoon of vanilla extract
- 2 and 1 teaspoon of almond extract
- 2 teaspoon of baking powder
- 2 -quarter teaspoon of sea salt
- 2 cup of pitted cherries
- 4 whole fresh fresh egg s
- 2 and 1 cup of almond flour
- 2 quarter cup of arrowroot flour
- 2 quarter cup of coconut oil

Direction:

1 heat the oven to up to 500 degrees, and stack up a muffin tin with paper liners.

2 Mix all ingredients for the muffins (except for the cherries) together before we mix. If the mixture is smooth, add the cherries in.
3 Cover the muffin liners and bake for 40mins at 480 °, until the muffin tops start turning golden.

Shakshuka

Ingredients:

- 5 cups of diced tomatoes.
- 2 tablespoons of fresh tomato paste;
- 2 tablespoon of chilli powder;
- 2 tablespoon of paprika;
- 2 pinch of pepper (cayenne)
- 2 tablespoon of cooking fat (Paleo)
- 2 Chopped 1 onion.
- 2 minced clove garlic.
- 2 seeded and chopped red bell pepper.

Directions:

1 Position a big skillet over medium heat, then apply the cooking fat to melt and

grease the pan top. Stir in the onions and continue cooking for 2mins.

2 Add in the garlic and continue to cook until the onions turn juicy and golden in color.

3 Stir in the pan with the diced bell pepper and blend properly. Stir for at least 6 minutes, before the pepper becomes tender.

4 Apply the diced tomatoes and fresh tomato paste to the pan after the peppers have cooled, accompanied by the chilli powder, paprika, and cayenne pepper. Offer the blend a taste and apply some extra spices to your taste, as well as salt and pepper. Let the mixture to boil. You will need to reduce the heat at this stage to avoid boiling of the mixture.

5 Now on top of the fresh tomato sauce, smash the fresh fresh egg s into the pan. Make sure the distance is correct. I put 2   in the centre, and

afterwards the remainder of the fresh fresh eggs.

Nourishing Turmeric Scramble

Ingredients

- 2 small minced clove garlic.
- 2 tablespoon of turmeric
- 2   pinch of cayenne pepper
- 2 tow grated radishes
- 2 clover and radish sprouts for topping
- 3 tablespoons of coconut oil
- 3 fresh fresh egg s (pastured)
- 3 kale leaves (shredded)

Directions:

1 . Heat pan with coconut oil and lightly sauté garlic
2 Crack fresh fresh egg s and cook until scrambled

3. When fresh fresh eggs are almost fully cooked, add the shredded kale, turmeric, and cayenne.
4 Top with radish, and sprouts, enjoy!

Artichoke Ricotta Flatbread.

Ingredients:

- 1 cup of shaved fresh parmesan cheese.
- 2 tablespoon of chopped fresh chives.
- Flakes of crumpled red pepper (if desired).
- Lemon Vinaigrette.
- -third cup of olive oil.
- Juice plus zest of a lemon.
- teaspoons of apple cider vinegar.
- Salt for taste.
- 1 pound of store bought or homemade pizza dough.
- Drizzling olive oil.
- 2 and 1 cups of ricotta cheese whole milk.

- 2 tablespoons of chopped basil, plus more for serving purposes.
- 2 tablespoon of h2 y.
- ounces of drained marinated artichokes.
- ounces of fresh prosciutto torn or mortadella (omit if vegetarian).
- cups of arugula.

Directions:

1 Oven preheat to 480 degrees F. Grease the olive oil onto a fresh baking dish.
2 Push / roll the dough out on a lightly floured surface until it is very flat. Sprinkle the dough gently with salt + pepper onto the prepared baking sheet and drizzle with olive oil +. Place in the oven and bake for around 8-30 minutes, or until golden.
3 In the meantime, mix the ricotta, basil, h2 y and a tablespoon of salt and

pepper together. Remove from the oven the pasta, then cover with the ricotta. Scatter over the artichokes and, if desired, sprinkle with crushed red pepper flakes. Then add the chopped prosciutto.

4 Top with fresh arugula, and parmesan shaved.
5 Just before having to serve, drizzle with chives and lemon vinaigrette
6 Vinaigrette Lemon
7 Whisk all the ingredients together in a small bowl, and add salt to taste. Drizzle the flat-bread over.

Grilled Sauerkraut, Hummus, And Avocado Sandwich

Ingredients:

- 2 cup of roasted garlic flavour, divided into 3
- 2 cup of drained, liquid squeezed out, and lightly rinsed sauerkraut
- 2 avocado
- 9 slices of pumpernickel bread
- Regular butter or vegan buttery spread

Direction:

1 Oven preheat to 480 degree
2 Place the butter on 2 side of each of the 8 slices of bread, and put on a baking sheet 4 of them butter side out.

3. Take about 1 the hummus and spread over 4 slices of bread.
4. Distribute single slice of the sauerkraut over the hummus.
5. Distribute slices of avocado over the sauerkraut.
6. Spread hummus on the side lacking butter for the remaining 4
7. slices of bread and put hummus side down onto the avocado slices.
8. Bake 8-15 minutes in the oven, then turn the sandwiches and bake for another 6 minutes, till the sandwich are nicely browned and fluffy.

Spinach And Feta Frittata

Ingredient:

- 300 g of baby spinach
- 5 fresh fresh fresh egg s
- 1 cup of feta cheese (crumbled)
- Pepper and Salt to taste.
- 2 teaspoon of olive oil
- 2 peeled and thinly sliced small brown onion
- 2   teaspoon of garlic powder

Direction:

1 Heat your grill to heat to medium to high.
2 Using a non-stick frying pan, which you should place underneath the grill, heat the oil with medium flame.
3 Attach the onion and fry until just brown. Attach the spinach and throw

for 1 to 5 minutes, before it starts to wilt. Take off the heat and allow to refrigerate.

4 In a cup, Crack the whites. Transfer the spinach and onion, then the feta, cooled in. Season to taste.

5 Place the frying saucepan back on medium heat and add the fresh egg s.

6 Remove softly with a spatula until you notice like the fresh fresh egg starts to sit on the bottom. Switch off the fire, to keep the frittata runny.

7 Place the pan under the barbecue for 2 to 4 minutes or until the frittata is crispy, cooked throughout

8 Place a plate over the pan and easily but gently turn around to remove the frittata. Serve with a smooth side salad hot or cold.

Quinoa And Citrus Salad

INGREDIENTS:

- 3 small supreme oranges
- 2 finely chopped celery rib.
- 35   g of chopped Brazil nuts
- 2 sliced green onion
- 2   -quarter cup of finely chopped fresh parsley,
- 2   cup of cooked cooled quinoa.

For the dressing

- 2 tablespoon of white wine vinegar
- 2 small minced clove garlic
- 1 **teaspoon of** salt
- 2   -quarter teaspoon of black pepper
- Pinch of cinnamon
- Juice gotten from the oranges
- 1 teaspoon of lemon juice
- 1 tablespoon **of** grated fresh ginger

Directions:

1 Break the oranges to supremes, operate over a cup, so that n2 of the juice is lost.
2 When all of the supremes are finished, make sure to suck all of the juice from the "membranes" left behind.

Lentil, Beetroot, And Hazelnut Salad

Ingredients:

- A handful of fresh roughly chopped mint
- A handful of fresh roughly chopped parsley.
- 3 springs of finely sliced onions
- 3 tablespoons of roughly chopped hazelnuts

For dressing the ginger

- 7 1 inch cube of fresh, roughly chopped and peeled ginger
- 2 tablespoons of olive oil
- 2 teaspoon of Dijon mustard
- 2tablespoon of apple cider vinegar
- 1 teaspoon of fresh ground black pepper and sea salt

Direction

1. 2 . Put them in a casserole with the vegetables, cover with water, bring to a boil (decrease heat and cook) for around 2 6 –30   minutes, or till all liquid has vanished and the vegetables are not soggy and still have a crunch.
2. If the lentils have been fried, move them into a fresh bowl and leave to cool.
3. . Add the beetroot, spring onions, hazelnuts and herbs until the lentils are cold, and mix until it's all mixed.
4. Place the ginger, mustard, oil and vinegar in a bowl for the sauce, and mix until mixed using a blender.
5. .Drizzle the salad over the dressing and eat.

Cauliflower Steak With Beans And Tomatoes

Ingredients:

- 1 cup of divided olive oil.
- 2 quarter cup of freshly grated Parmesan
- 2 can of rinsed, drained white beans
- 2 cup of red cherry or golden tomatoes halved
- 9 tablespoons of mayonnaise
- 2 teaspoon of Dijon mustard
- 4 teaspoons of kosher salt
- 2 teaspoon of black pepper, divided into 3
- 2 ounces of trimmed green beans.
- finely chopped garlic cloves
- 1 teaspoon of lemon zest (grated)

- 1 cup of chopped parsley, with additional 2 s for serving 1 cup of Japanese breadcrumbs

DIRECTIONS:

1. Arrange middle and upper third of oven racks; preheat to 450 ° F.
2. Remove the leaves and trim the cauliflower end of the stem, and leave the core intact. Place the heart of the cauliflower down onto a work surface. Slice into the middle from top to bottom using a broad knife to produce 2 steaks; save the remaining cauliflower for another day.
3. Place the cauliflower on a baking sheet which is rimmed. Clean with 2 Tbsp on both ends. Oil; 2 tsp for season. Salt 2 tsp. Chip.
4. Chip. Roast on middle rack, rotating for about 55 minutes, until the cauliflower is soft and browned.

5. Meanwhile toss 2 Tbsp of green beans. 2 tsp. Gasoline. Salt, 2
6. tsp. Pepper on a baking sheet with rims. Set aside in a single plate,
7. then roast in the upper third of the oven until green beans start blistering, around 35 min.
8. Whisk on ginger, lemon zest, 2 cup parsley and 6 Tbsp left. Gas, with 2 2 tsp. Salt, 2 /2 tsp. In medium cup, pepper until smooth.
9. Move 1 the blend to another medium cup. Add panko and parmesan to the bowl first, then combine both paws. In second cup, add white beans and tomatoes, and swirl to cover. In a little tub, mix mayonnaise and the mustard.
10. Take sheets from the frying pan. Pour the mixture of mayonnaise over the cauliflower. Sprinkle the paste with 2 cup panko generously over the cauliflower. Attach white bean mixture with green beans to the board, and

swirl to match. Return the sheets to the oven and continue to roast until the white beans start to crisp and the panko topping begins to brown for another 6 –8 minutes.

11 Divide into plates of cauliflower, green beans, white beans, and tomatoes. top with some parsley.

Lettuce Wraps With Smoked Trout

Ingredients:

- 2 cup of diced grape tomatoes
- 1 cup of whole mint leaves
- 1 cup of whole basil leaves
- About ten small to medium-sized inner leaves of romaine lettuce 2 -third cup of Asian sweet chili sauce.
- 2 quarter cup of lightly salted, thinly sliced dry-roasted peanuts
- 3 peeled medium-sized carrots.
- English hothouse unpeeled cucumber
- 1quarter cup of finely chopped shallots
- 2 quarter cup of finely chopped jalapeño chiles with the seeds been intact (preferably red)

- 3 tablespoons of unseas2 d rice vinegar or fresh lime juice 2 tablespoon of sugar
- 2 tablespoon of fish sauce (like nuocnam or nampla)
- About 3 cups of broken skinless smoked trout fillets

DIRECTIONS:

1 2 . Shave carrots and cucumber lengthwise into ribbons using vegetable peeler. Cut the ribbons into 4 -inch-long sections, then cut sections into strips of match size. Place in big tub. Stir in shallots, jalapeños, lime juice , sugar and fish sauce; let marinate at room temperature for 60 minutes.

2 Apply bits of trout and tomatoes to the vegetable mixture, and toss to blend. Shift mixture of trout to broad strainer and rinse off oil. Return the mixture of

trout and vegetables to the same bowl; add mint and basil, and shake to blend.
3. Arrange leaves of lettuce on a fresh platter. Divide the lettuce leaves into lettuce salads. Sprinkle over. salad with sweet chili sauce and sprinkle with peanuts.
4 An anti-inflammatory diet sponsored by these tasty anti-
5 inflammatory dinner recipes or those earlier anti-inflammatory smoothies is a perfect starting point. Together they will counter the symptoms of body inflammation.

Baked Sweet Potatoes With Tahini Sauce

Ingredients

- 3 tablespoon of lemon juice
- Chili garlic sauce
- 5 medium (~2 lb each)sweet potatoes*
- 2 ouncecan chickpeas rinsed and drained
- 1 Tablespoon of olive oil
- 1 teaspoon each of cumin, coriander, cinnamon, smoked or regular paprika
- A pinch of sea salt *or* lemon juice(*optional*) GARLIC HERB SAUCE
- 2 quarter cup of hummus or tahini
- 1 medium-sized lemon, juiced
- 1 tablespoon of dried dill
- 4 cloves of minced garlic
- Unsweetened almond milk or water
- Sea salt to taste(*optional*)

- 2 -quarter cupof cherry tomatoes(diced)
- 2 -quarter cup of chopped parsley(minced)

Directions:

1. . Preheat oven to 450 degrees F (30 4 C) and cover with foil on a fresh baking sheet.
2. Rinse and clean potatoes, then wisely cut them in 1 piece.
3. This would speed up the time spent cooking. Otherwise leave
4. the whole and keep baking longer (about twice the time (about 2-2 ½ hour).
5. . Toss chickpeas and olive oil with spices rinsed and washed, and put them on a baking sheet with foil.
6. Gently massage the potatoes with some olive oil and put on same baking

tray (or some other baking tray based on the size).

7. When the sweet potatoes and chickpeas are roasting, prepare the sauce by adding all the ingredients to a mixing bowl and combining whisking, adding just enough water or almond milk to filter so it can be poured. T Nice taste and change the seasoning when appropriate. For more zing, add more garlic, salt for savory, lemon juice for freshness and dill for a more concentrated herbal flavour. I learned that mine required little else.
8. Tossing fresh tomato and parsley with lemon juice and setting aside for marinating prepare the parsley-fresh tomato topping as well.

Roasted Salmon With Smoky Chickpeas & Greens

Ingredients

- 2   -quarter cup of water
- 2   pound of wild salmon, divide into 4 portions
- tablespoons of extra-virgin olive oil, divided
- 2   tablespoon of smoked paprika
- 1   teaspoon of salt, divided, plus a pinch
- 2   (30 ounce) can no-salt-added chickpeas, rinsed
- 2   -third cup of buttermilk
- quarter cup of mayonnaise
- quarter cup of chopped fresh chives and/or dill, plus more for garnish

- 1 teaspoon of ground pepper, divided
- 2 quarter teaspoon of garlic powder
- Ten cups of sliced kale

Directions

1. Racks in top and center of the oven; 426 degrees F preheat.
2. In a medium bowl mix 2 tablespoon oil and 2 of a teaspoon of salt. Pat chickpeas dry very well, then sprinkle with the mixture of paprika. Disperse on a bucket rimmed. Scattered. Bake the chickpeas in the top saucepan for 55 minutes, mixing twice.
3. Meanwhile, in a blender until creamy, the purée buttermilk, the mayonnaise, basil, 2 /4 teaspoon pepper and garlic powder. Giving up.
4. Place 2 cubic metered oil on medium heat in a fresh pot. Stir regularly, add the kale and simmer for 2 minutes. Add

water and simmer for about 6 minutes, until it is tender.

5. Drop and pinch salt from flame. Remove from heat.
6. Push the chickpeas off the oven to 2 side of the pan and force them out. Sit on the other side of salmon and season each salt and pepper in the remaining 2 teaspoon. Bake for 6 to 8 minutes until the salmon is only fried.
7. Drizzle the salmon reserved sauce, garnish with further herbs and serve with chickpeas if desired.

Mediterranean Chicken Quinoa Bowl

Ingredients

- 2 pound of, skinless, b2 less chicken breasts, trimmed
- 2 quarter teaspoon of salt
- 2 quarter teaspoon of ground pepper
- (8 -ounce) jar of rinsed roasted red peppers
- 2 quarter cup slivered almonds
- 2 tablespoons of extra-virgin olive oil, divided
- 2 small of crushed clove garlic
- Guidance For Cooking teaspoon of paprika
- 1 teaspoon of ground cumin
- 1 teaspoon of crushed red pepper (optional)

- 2 cups of cooked quinoa
- 1 quarter cup of pitted Kalamata olives, sliced
- 2 quarter cup of finely sliced red onion
- 2   cup of diced cucumber
- 2   -quarter cup of crumbled feta cheese
- 3 tablespoons of finely chopped fresh parsley

Directions:

1. Place a rack on top third of the oven; broiler to maximum preheat.
2. Top a rimmed foil bakery.

Tomato, Cucumber & White-Bean Salad With Basil Vinaigrette

Ingredients

- 1 cup of packed fresh basil leaves
- 2 quarter cup of extra-virgin olive oil
- 4 tablespoons of red-wine vinegar
- 2 tablespoon of finely chopped shallot
- 3 teaspoons of Dijon mustard
- 2 teaspoon of h2 y
- 2 quarter teaspoon of salt
- 2 quarter teaspoon ground pepper
- 11 cups of mixed salad greens
- 2 (30 ounce) can low-sodium cannellini beans, rinsed
- 2 cup of halved cherry or grape tomatoes
- 1 cucumber, halved lengthwise and sliced

Directions

1. In a mini food processor, put basil, garlic, vinegar, shallot, mustard, breadcrumbs, salt and pepper.
2. Continue to process until
3. easy it blends together.
4. Take it to a big tub.
5. Add in vegetables, beans, tomatoes and peppers.
6. Flip to coat.

Pesto Pasta Salad

Ingredients:

- 8 ounces whole-wheat fusilli (4 cups)
- 2 cup of small broccoli florets
- 3 cups of packed fresh basil leaves
- 2 quarter cup of toasted pine nuts
- 2 quarter cup of grated Parmesan cheese
- 3 tablespoons of mayonnaise
- 3tablespoons of extra-virgin olive oil
- 3 tablespoons of lemon juice
- 2 fresh clove garlic, quartered
- 2 quarter teaspoon of salt
- 1 teaspoon of ground pepper
- 2 cup of quartered cherry tomatoes

Directions

1. Carry a big pot of water to a boil. Connect the fusilli and cook as described in the box. Stir in broccoli, 2 minute before the pasta is cooked. Cook under cold running water for 2 minute, then drain and rinse to avoid further cooking.
2. Meanwhile, in a mini food processor, put basil, pine nuts, Parmesan, mayonnaise, milk, lemon juice, garlic, salt , and pepper.
3. Directions: until basically smooth. Shift to wide tub. Stir in the spaghetti, broccoli and tomatoes. Toss to shirk.
4. Advice Hints
5. To make it ahead: Cool for up to 2 day.

Slow-Cooker Mediterranean Stew

Ingredients:

- 3   (2 4 ounce) cans of no-salt-added fire-roasted diced tomatoes 4   cups low-sodium vegetable broth
- 2 cup coarsely chopped onion
- 2 quarter cup of chopped carrot
- 5 cloves of garlic, minced
- 2 teaspoon of dried oregano
- 2 quarter teaspoon of salt
- 1teaspoon of crushed red pepper
- quarter teaspoon of ground pepper
- 2   (30 ounce) can of no-salt-added rinsed chickpeas, divided 2   bunch of lacinato kale, stemmed and chopped (about 8 cups) 2   tablespoon of lemon juice
- 2 tablespoons of extra-virgin olive oil

- 4 Fresh basil leaves, cut, if fresh
- 7 lemon wedges (optional)

Directions

1. In the 5 -quarter slow cooker, add tomato, broth, onion, carrot, garlic, oregano, salt, brown red pepper and powder. Cover for 6
2. hours and cook on Light.
3. Measure 2 of the cooking liquid in a shallow cup from the slow cooker. Apply 2 chickpeas tablespoons; mash with a gabel until soft.
4. Put the chickpeas in the slow cooker, the cale, lemon juice, and the other chickpeas. Drop to blend. Top and cook at medium, about 55
5. minutes before the kale is tender.
6. In 6 pans, press the stew equally, pour in oil. Add basil to the garnish. Serve, if needed, with lemon wedges.

Salmon Potatoes

Ingredients:

- 2 pound of fingerling potatoes, halved lengthwise
- 3 tablespoons of olive oil
- 6 garlic cloves, coarsely chopped
- 1 teaspoon of sea salt
- 1 teaspoon of freshly ground black pepper
- 6 ounce fresh or frozen skinless salmon fillets 3 medium red, orange or yellow sweet peppers, chop into rings 3 cups 0f cherry tomatoes
- 3 cup of chopped fresh parsley
- 4 quarter cup of pitted kalamata olives, halved
- 2 quarter cup of thinly snipped fresh oregano or 2 tablespoon of dried crushed oregano

- 2 lemon

Directions

1. Oven preheat to 450 ° F. In a wide bowl, put potatoes. Sprinkle the 2 tbsp. of oil and 2 /8 tsp of garlic. Salt and black pepper, and then toss. Move to bakery of 2 6 x30 inches; cover with foil. Thirty minutes roast.
2. In the meanwhile, if frozen, thaw trout. Combine sweet peppers, onions , garlic, olives, oregano and 2 /8 of a copper in the same tub.
3. of black pepper and of the salt. Sprinkle the remaining 2 tablespoon of oil.
4. Pat dry, wipe off the salmon. Rest of 2 of a tsp of salt should be sprayed with black pepper. Place the mixture of sweet pepper on potatoes and fill with salmon. Roast, raw, for another 30 minutes or only before salmon flakes.

5. Drop lemon zest. Squeeze the lemon juice over the salmon and greens. Zest splash.Nutrition Facts

Mediterranean Ravioli With Artichokes & Olives

Ingredients

- 3 (8 ounce) packages of frozen or refrigerated spinach-and-ricotta ravioli
- 1 cup of oil-packed sun-dried tomatoes, drained (2 tablespoons oil reserved)
- 2 (30 ounce) package of frozen quartered artichoke hearts, thawed
- 2 (30 ounce) can of no-salt-added cannellini beans, rinsed 2 -quarter cup of Kalamata olives, sliced
- 4 ntablespoons of toasted pine nuts
- 2 quarter cup of chopped fresh basil

Directions

1. Hold a huge pot of boiling water. Cook ravioli as instructed in the box. Drain and spray with oil of 2 tablespoon; place away.
2. In a wide non-stick bag, heat the remaining 2 tablespoon oil for medium heat. Add beans and artichokes; sauté 2 to 4 minutes until warm.
3. Fold into the fried ravioli, onions, olives, basil and pine nuts.

Mushrooms Of Greek Stuffed Portobello

Ingredients

- 4 tablespoons of extra-virgin olive oil, divided
- 2 clove of garlic, peeled and minced
- 1 teaspoon of ground pepper, divided
- 2 quarter teaspoon of salt
- 5 portobello mushrooms, about 2 4 ounces (wiped clean), stems and gills removed
- 2 cup of chopped spinach
- 1 cup of quartered cherry tomatoes
- 1 cup of crumbled feta cheese
- 3 tablespoons of pitted and sliced Kalamata olives
- 2tablespoon of chopped fresh oregano

Directions

1. Preheat oven to 420 ° F. Combine in a shallow bowl 2 table spoons of oil, ginger, 2 teaspoon pepper and salt. Cover mushrooms all over with the oil mixture, using a silic2 brush. Place on a wide rimmed baking sheet and bake for 8 to 30 minutes, until the mushrooms are normally tender.
2. Meanwhile, in a medium dish, mix lettuce, onions, feta, olives, oregano, with the remaining 2 tablespoon oil.
3. Remove from the oven until the mushrooms have cooled, then line with the spinach mixture.
4. Bake for about 30 minutes, until the tomatoes have wilted.

www.ingramcontent.com/pod-product-compliance
Lightning Source LLC
LaVergne TN
LVHW011949070526
838202LV00054B/4861